Diagnosing & Treating Common Nutritional Deficiencies

When the Body is Lacking Essential Nutrients

By: James M. Lowrance © 2010

TABLE OF CONTENTS:

INTRODUCTION

Nutritional deficiencies have increased in frequency worldwide. Even the most industrialized countries in the world are seeing more cases of deficiency in vitamins, minerals, proteins, electrolytes and other essential elements in their populations. What is responsible for these imbalances in nutrients? A major factor in the more industrialized countries of the world is "inappropriate diet". With the increase in manufacture of junk foods over the past five decades and especially over the past three, people are getting fewer foods with nutritional value, in their diets. Some brands of purified water being used exclusively as drinking water, in attempt to eliminate toxins such as excessive fluoride may be lacking essential minerals and electrolytes at the same time.

This has led to an increase in the trend for using nutritional supplements, to help offset the harmful effects of inappropriate diet. Some advocates for better health, are also seeing the need to add mineral-electrolyte drops to purified drinking water for revitalization.

Certainly safe, quality-manufactured supplements of these types are highly beneficial under the proper circumstances. The fact is however, that healthy supplements are less-effective, in cases of bad diet and lifestyle practices.

Nutrients need a healthy body to work properly in and unhealthy lifestyle practices, such as inadequate sleep, lack of proper exercise, excessive intake of junk foods and inadequate intake of nutritional foods can seriously hinder the effectiveness of natural health supplements. This is due to the fact that the different types of nutrients work in a loop – so that they compliment the purpose of one another (synchronicity).

When one nutrient becomes deficient, this can cause imbalances in others. Low levels of the mineral-electrolytes; phosphate (hypophosphatemia) and/or calcium (hypocalcemia) can be a direct result of vitamin D deficiency for example.

It is important to determine if there are nutrients that are specifically deficient, so that they are not excluded from a supplement regimen.

Also, if a particular nutrient is already at proper levels in the body or at high-normal or even at levels that would be flagged-high when blood lab tested, adding more to a person's system, could cause a toxic reaction. One example of over-supplementation would be that of someone taking a dose of iron each day that exceeds the RDA (Recommended Daily Allowance) when they already have sufficient levels in their body. This can potentially result in a condition of iron-overload called "hemochromatosis". This condition causes iron to be stored in vital organs in dangerously high amounts, which can lead to damage and eventual shut-down of them (i.e. the liver, kidneys and heart). These facts point to the importance of lab testing, symptom-monitoring and receiving advice from a qualified physician when possible to avoid causing further nutritional imbalances. These are some of the aspects I will be addressing in the chapters that follow.

This information-resource is not intended to be extensive or complete in regard to all nutritional deficiencies that exist and so I will be addressing some of the more common types and the treatments that are administered to resolve them.

I will also include is a comprehensive list of vitamins, minerals and electrolytes and the symptoms that occur with deficiencies of these essential nutrients in "CHAPTER FIVE". It is important that suspected deficiencies are confirmed medically by blood lab testing and proper evaluation by a medical professional.

CHAPTER ONE:

Causes of Nutritional Deficiencies

Junk Foods

Even in the decades of the 1950s and 1960s, there was far more consumption per-person, of fruits, vegetables, nuts and grains. This began changing even more dramatically in the 1970s, with snack food companies increasing their product and promotion for lines of cookies, candies, pastries, pies, cakes and soft drinks. This is causing a lack in the diet of both "macronutrients" (protiens) and "micronutrients" (vitamins) in a large portion of our population. The stimulant effects of these junk foods and from the caffeine in soft drinks, is often used as a substitute for the steady energy levels that can be obtained through adequate intake of nutritional foods.

The incidence of obesity has climbed dramatically over the past two decades as well, due to diets containing a high level of these simple carbohydrates as opposed to more complex carbohydrates containing essential nutrients, to keep the body healthy.

As a result, cases of metabolic diseases and health disorders have also increased dramatically, including diabetes, fatty liver disease and metabolic syndrome (a pre-diabetic condition). It is also important to note that people who follow strict vegan diets (vegetarian) will sometimes lack intake of essential nutrients found in fish, poultry and beef. If one is determined to follow a strict vegan-ism regimen, this may increase the need for nutrient supplementation and closer monitoring for any symptoms of nutritional deficiency that may develop over time. Yearly blood retesting of essential nutrients (i.e. the major vitamins, protein levels and complete blood counts) becomes important in these type cases as well.

Environmental Toxins

Some medical trend observers have also cited "environmental toxins" as a factor involved in less-absorption of nutrients in the human body. With more pollutants and toxins being introduced into our environment, due to the increase in manufacturing of products of all types and with the increase of additives and preservatives in manufactured foods, nutrients are in-essence being blocked in the body.

Enrichment of nutrients in foods that are grown is also being hindered due to these environmental changes.

Heavy metals and toxic chemicals such as mercury are being found in patients by their doctors that have been absorbed into their systems from things such as silver tooth fillings(amalgam) or from plastic drinking bottles (bisphenol). These metals and chemicals can hinder the ability of nutrients to do their job in keeping the body healthy. The increase in toxins also serves to confuse the immune system, which has given rise in the incidence of autoimmune diseases and immunocompromised states of health according to some medical sources.

Malabsorption Syndromes

Other vitamin deficient people, are suffering from "malabsorption syndromes", which means their bodies are not properly absorbing vitamins from things consumed in their diets. For some of these people, they are lacking proper amounts of enzymes in the body that help them to extract and utilize vitamins or to break-down proteins, fats or sugars (glucose).

This process must occur so that these nutrients can be transferred into the cells of the body for proper energy (hydrolysis) and to maintain the strength of muscle, bones, cartilage, skin, and blood . If malabsorption is that of fats that are consumed not being broken-down and used for energy, the body will instead pass these fats, rather than absorbing and metabolizing them and the person will experience greasy stools and/or frequent diarrhea.

The same is true of bowel diseases such as Crohn's disease (autoimmune) and Celiac disease (intolerance for gluten in the diet), which cause severe diarrhea and eventual intestinal damage if not treated. A type of malabsorption that does not always result in bowel symptoms but that leads to weakened red blood cells is "pernicious anemia". This disorder of nutritional deficiency is caused by lack of a protein-enzyme in the digestive tract called "intrinsic factor", a substance that extracts and utilized vitamin B12 from things consumed in the diet. In this case, the immune system recognizes this key enzyme as an intruder in the body and begins to destroy it, causing the development of this potentially severe and even life-threatening type of anemia.

Certain types of viral infections such as "Helicobacter Pylori" and overgrowth of diploid funguses such as "Candida Albicans" can also result in severe digestive disorders and malabsorption of essential nutrients.

A less-severe type of autoimmune digestive disorder is "Autoimmune Atrophic Gastritis", an inflammatory disease of the stomach-lining (mucosa) that occurs in older adults and in people with other types of autoimmune diseases (i.e. thyroid autoimmunity, rheumatoid arthritis and Lupus). In the case of this digestive disease, malabsorption occurs due to destruction of the stomach lining and atrophy of the stomach (shrinkage), resulting in a loss of ability for proper digestion and nutritional metabolism to occur.

Another factor in malabsorption syndromes is imbalances in the level of hydrochloric stomach acid (digestive juices). Achlorhydria is the term for low stomach acid and this condition can prevent proper break-down of foods so that proper digestion of them can occur and nutrients can be extracted for use in the body.

Rarely, over-use of acid-blocking drugs to treat acid indigestion and GERD (Gastroesophageal Reflux Disease), can cause excessive lowering of stomach acid or the body may simply be producing inadequate amounts of this digestive agent.

Intestinal Parasites

While it is not often recognized, parasitic infections are not uncommon in industrialized countries, including the USA and when they occur, they can cause bowel disease that includes nutrient malabsorption as a symptom.

Parasites can be present in certain types of consumed foods, such as fruits and vegetables that are not properly washed, meats that are undercooked, water that has not been purified and from improper hygiene – especially the failure to wash one's hands before handling and preparing food.

Parasites can also be transmitted to humans through pets or from the feces of them that makes its way into their homes.

Common and less-common parasites in the USA for example, include Enterobius vermicularis (pinworms), Giardia lamblia (microscopic parasite), Ancylostoma duodenale (nematode worm), Necator americanus (hookworm), Entamoeba histolytica (protozoan ameba). In addition to digestive disease, some parasites can also result in liver damage, which demonstrates the importance in protective measures against contracting them and early diagnosis and treatment when infections with them do occur.

Liver Problems

Yet others, who suffer vitamin deficiencies, are experiencing types of liver diseases that prevent the organ from doing its job in converting fats, proteins and sugars into energy cells. The liver infact also plays a role in hormone-synthetization, meaning it takes precursor hormones and converts them into essential end-hormones, with the help of other organs in the body, including the kidneys. Types of hepatitis (inflammatory liver disease) can result in liver malfunction as can problems with the bile ducts in the liver that normally transport bile to the intestines, so that fat and fat-soluable vitamins can be absorbed by the body.

In some cases of bile duct disease, an autoimmune attack is directed at this part of the liver, causing damage and scarring, also referred-to as "biliary sclerosis". Alcohol abuse and certain types of drugs of both the prescribed and illegal types can result in liver damage over time as well; in fact excessive use of some types of over-the-counter drugs can also result in liver damage, in some cases, leading to malabsorption of nutrients.

In the chapters that follow I will address some of the more-common nutritional deficiencies that are being experienced and treatments that are medically administered or self-administered to correct them and to prevent them from re-occurring.

CHAPTER TWO:

My Personal Experience with Vitamin Deficiencies

I was diagnosed with autoimmune thyroiditis (Hashimoto's disease) and hypothyroidism in year-2003. My thyroid hormone therapy never seemed to relieve my symptoms of fatigue, muscle weakness and general body aches, so I assumed for all that time that I had a comorbid condition such as Chronic Fatigue Syndrome and/or Fibromyalgia. While there are great MDs out there, most I went-to in the area I reside-in, were ill-informed on many things, such as nutritional deficiencies. I was not ordered blood tests that could have diagnosed factors involved in my eventual development of peripheral neuropathies (PN) much sooner, so that I could have received treatments to prevent permanent nerve damage.

Early in the year 2010, I finally began demanding blood tests of vitamin levels due to ongoing muscle weakness in my arms and legs (myopathy).

These symptoms worsened but were very slowly progressing over an approximate ten year span of time. I also began to develop some deep aching in my limbs and in the heels of my feet that became significantly painful. I also began developing tingling, burning and aching, sensations in them that would flare much worse after walking. I also began to experience a degree of stiffness in my feet when getting up from sleeping or even after sitting for only a few minutes at a time. Carpal tunnel symptoms began to worsen in my hands and wrists but were more prominent on my right side (my dominant one).

My vitamin D level was the first to be found deficient via blood lab testing @ "17" (range 20 to 100) and afterward my B12 was found in the "insufficiency" range (low-normal but not flagged low), @ "374" (range 600 to 1100). Treatment for these did not relieve my symptoms as well as expected, so I requested to be referred to a neurologist and he tested me for more vitamin deficiencies, including B6 and E levels. My vitamin E ended up being my most severe deficiency, coming in on my blood result, @ "0.4" (range 3.0 to 15.8).

I searched reputable online medical sources and found information stating that E-deficiency causes "certain neurological damage" (not a possible but a definite). I believe my thyroid autoimmunity, combined with my nutritional deficiencies, is the cause of my peripheral neuropathies, in fact even common sense revealed this to me. My neurologist had me to undergo further, extensive blood testing and I was found to be negative for muscle wasting diseases (i.e. CK and other muscle enzymes tested in normal range). I was also found to be negative for Lyme disease and Celiac disease. My EMG/Nerve Conduction testing showed abnormal readings (low amplitude) in a number of my nerves.

My vitamin deficiencies can explain a great deal in regard to symptoms I developed but vitamin replacement therapy for them has so-far not completely corrected my peripheral neuropathy. This is likely due to the fact that a degree of irreversible nerve damage occurred from longstanding vitamin E deficiency. My symptoms have however improved a great deal, from my pre vitamin replacement state and further recovery may occur over time.

I do not have fat malabsorption or liver/biliary involvement in my deficiencies, which were ruled-out with extensive blood testing, so apparently these are idiopathic deficiencies (no determinable cause). A major blood test that helped rule the disease out in my case was to detect Antimitochondrial Antibodies (AMA) which was negative.

One possible explanation is that my deficiencies may be directly associated with my autoimmune thyroid disease. Diabetes was also found to be negative via my lab evaluations, which I was thankful to have ruled out. My low vitamin E has been replaced via therapy as previously mentioned and is now in the upper-normal range. This is the treatment from which I saw the most significant improvement in my neurological symptoms, which reveals to me that in my case, the low vitamin E was the one most detrimental to my neurological health.

It is also possible, as I have learned through medical search, that my development of autoimmune thyroid disease is related to my vitamin D deficiency.

It has been found in medical research studies, to cause immune system problems in patients who are deficient in the vitamin. There have been studies showing that it places people with both deficiency (blood-level readings of 20 ng/mL and below) and insufficiency (blood-level readings of 30 ng/mL and below) at risk for autoimmune diseases and other chronic and inflammatory diseases, including those affecting the thyroid gland (i.e. Graves' disease and Hashimoto's thyroiditis).

Autoimmune thyroiditis very rarely goes into remission or I should say is rarely ever reversed but is usually a life-long disease. Replacing low vitamin D levels is very important but will not cure the disease, although it may prevent its development in susceptible individuals. So far no treatments have been found to cure autoimmunity of any kind that is already present although patients with Graves' disease can see hyperthyroidism permanently resolved with thyroid removal or ablation of their thyroid glands with radioactive iodine. They do afterward have to be treated permanently with thyroid hormone replacement as hypothyroidism develops once the thyroid has been removed.

One thing that does help reduce thyroid antibody levels, the immune cells that cause these diseases according to medical research studies, is supplementation with "selenium" at the recommended dose on the manufacturer's label. Other than this treatment which can reduce but not eliminate thyroid antibodies, there is no cure for thyroid autoimmunity itself. If there were a cure or one is developed at some point in the future, I will certainly have the treatment administered for my own Hashimoto's thyroiditis.

Some sources I searched in regard to the prescription-only, high-potency form of vitamin D called "Drisdol" (my prescribed treatment for D-deficiency) state that it is a commonly prescribed "D2" replacement vitamin. I read the information on my prescription bottle and it says "Generic for: DRISDOL". It also states on the label: "50,000UNT" and "The mfg: BRENC" (apparently an abbreviation for the company that makes it). Some sources state that vitamin D deficiency needs to be treated with a "D3" supplement rather than with the D2 type of replacement, for better improvement.

The real proof of its effectiveness for each individual however, will be symptom-relief experienced and blood retest levels, to monitor the treatment.

I will be retested on my "25(OH) D" level (medical lab term for vitamin D in the blood) at regular intervals of about once a year, following my initial labs showing corrected levels. If I remember correctly the blood test shows both D2 – the supplemented level coming into the body and the D3 – the natural converted level (I request copies of all labs I have done).

While my original deficiency reading was "17" as mentioned previously, even a level of 30 is considered "insufficiency" and I believe they prefer to see the level increased to at least 50 or above, which is about mid-range, on up to higher-normal values.

Should this Vitamin D brand not correct my deficient levels properly, as reflected in follow-up blood retests, I will ask for a change to D3 supplementation that the sources I mentioned previously, are stating is superior for correcting deficiency.

If I were to make a statement regarding my case, I would hope that it would be to present a case for the importance in being blood-tested for vitamin deficiencies. I believe it is possible that had my vitamin E deficiency not been discovered, I would have eventually succumbed to irreversible neurological damage and possible death, with my level of the vitamin having reached such a severely deficient state. I remember at one point, the muscles in my right hand felt as if they literally gave-out on me as I worked on replacing the faucets on a bathroom sink.

This required me to use hand tools and after using my grip repeatedly, the muscles in my hand and upper arm stopped functioning. I was also experiencing a feeling of general un-wellness and I remarked to my wife that I literally felt as if I was slowly dying and that I needed to see a medical specialist who could get to the bottom of the cause of my illness.

Yes, nutrition deficiencies can become fatal if they become severe enough and there is a failure in treating them.

The human body simply cannot survive or function properly without proper nutrition and some nutrients, including vitamins E and B12 are essential for healthy blood and nerves. If a patient is seeing a doctor who is reluctant to order blood testing for vitamin deficiencies, they should ask for a referral to a doctor who is willing to order the proper lab tests or they should immediately seek a new doctor on their own.

When I was originally diagnosed with autoimmune hypothyroidism in late 2003 and early 2004, one of the first doctors I was seeing for treatment would not agree to order blood tests of my vitamin levels. I requested testing due to my thyroid hormone replacement therapy, failing to restore my health to a reasonably improved level. I specifically mentioned to this doctor that I felt I was experiencing a vitamin deficiency. I made this mention to members of my family even prior to this discussion with my doctor. He replied by saying that vitamin deficiencies were rare and that vitamins usually do not mean a great deal.

This is a shocking reply for a doctor to make and has a great deal to do with my reason for becoming proactive in my health care and in my becoming a patent advocate in helping to generally inform fellow-patients.

<u>CHAPTER THREE:</u>

The Vitamin-D Deficiency Epidemic

Not only do medical sources state that vitamin D levels must be adequate in the body for calcium and magnesium to work properly but vitamin D is an essential vitamin, that some medical research experts actually refer-to as a steroid hormone because of its other varied, far-reaching and essential effects in the human body. It is now recognized by medical research groups as a vitamin that is found more commonly deficient in the general population than was formerly believed. Vitamin D makes calcium work properly in the bones, to keep them healthy but it also plays a role in keeping muscles operating properly, including the heart.

This essential vitamin has also been shown in medical research studies, to help prevent the onset of type II – adult onset diabetes. Vitamin D is also essential in keeping the emotions balanced and the nervous system functioning properly. It has also been found in medical research studies, to help prevent cancer from developing in those whose levels of the vitamin stay at adequate or optimal levels.

A healthy diet and plenty of sunshine can help to keep vitamin D replenished in the body but for some individuals, their bodies do not properly absorb the vitamin in their digestive tracts due to conditions of malabsorption that can be inherited or acquired (caused by a disease process). Some individuals also fail to get a proper amount of sunshine, which causes vitamin D to be produced on the surface of the skin and absorbed into the body but is only one major source we receive it from.

Foods that are rich in vitamin D include the following:

- Eggs
- Liver and Beef
- Salmon and Sardines
- Mackerel and Tuna
- Milk and Yogurt - vitamin D-fortified
- Orange juice
- Mushrooms
- Cod liver oil

Supplementation via a daily dose of vitamin D can help to assure that one is receiving proper levels.

The U.S. RDA (recommended daily allowance) of vitamin D for children above the age of 12-months and for adults is 50 mcg (2,000 IU) daily. Some medical research groups however, believe that this RDA should be revised and should be set much higher to better protect against heart disease and later-life bone loss diseases such as osteoporosis.

A condition called "rickets" is the main symptom of vitamin D deficiency in children, which causes bone deformities, such as bowed legs and a lack of skeletal growth. In adults, bones also become softened due to deficiency, which can cause them to fracture easily. Adults will often experience pain that radiates from the bones as well, muscle weakness and possible neurological symptoms including peripheral neuropathies when they lack proper levels of vitamin D.

If vitamin D deficiency is suspected, it is important that a qualified medical doctor is consulted. A simple blood test called the "25-hydroxyvitamin D" (also called "25-hydroxycholecalciferol) can determine whether or not vitamin D is at an adequate level.

If it is found deficient, supplementation at replacement doses that are usually much higher than the RDA can be administered. When deficiency is not present, the RDA of vitamin D can be safely taken to prevent deficiency from developing.

Can Getting Ample Sunlight Still Leave You Vitamin D Deficient?

(Note: The body absorbs vitamins through the diet, by way of the digestive system and through the skin via activation by sunlight, which are responses regulated by the involuntary nervous system. Vitamin D is essential for proper nerve function as mentioned above.)

You can still be low on vitamin D, even with getting plenty of sunshine because much of what the body needs also comes through the diet and while many foods have vitamin D in them; a person can fail to absorb it, due to a number of possible digestive problems. People with autoimmune gastro-intestinal disorders, such as Crohn's Disease, Celiac Disease and Pernicious Anemia, can have problems absorbing vitamins from things in their diets.

This is because they lack the intestinal enzymes that are needed to do so, due to them being destroyed by auto-antibodies that come from the immune system. Chronic diarrhea, that occurs for any reason can also cause failure to absorb vitamins such as D and the other major nutrients. A condition called "malabsorption syndrome" can as well and this one occurs due to gallstones obstructing the bile duct that goes from the gallbladder to the liver or from the duct being destroyed by autoimmune process (biliary cirrhosis). The malabsorption can also be due to a person not being able to absorb fat from the diet (fat malabsorption syndrome) and since some vitamins, such as D, E, A and K are "fat soluble", if fat is not properly absorbed from the diet, the vitamins have no carrier substance to take them into the cells of the body.

For these reasons, adequate amounts of sunshine may still not be enough to prevent vitamin D deficiency and when it occurs, high-dose oral supplementation is required to replace levels back to normal range and afterward; the highest RDA of vitamin D will likely be required for the rest of one's life.

CHAPTER FOUR:

Pernicious Anemia – Vitamin B12 Deficiency

Pernicious anemia is an autoimmune disorder and is more common in patients who already suffer from other types of autoimmune diseases. This brief chapter can help one to recognize this potentially serious type of anemia.

Symptoms of pernicious anemia are those of other types with the addition of possible neurological symptoms in severe cases.

All anemic conditions result in low or inadequate red blood cell counts, causing the patient to have tired blood. This simply means that the red blood cells are inadequate to carry sufficient amounts of oxygen to the cells of the body for energy and the same is true of pernicious anemia.

The general symptoms of anemia are:

• weakness
• headache
• dizziness
• pale complexion ...

...

- fast heartbeat (tachycardia)
- shortness of breath
- difficulty concentrating
- cold extremities

People with pernicious anemia are also at risk of developing neurological symptoms if the condition worsens due to non-treatment or delayed treatment.

Symptoms involving nerves may include the following.

- numbness
- burning and tingling in the legs, arms, feet and hands
- loss of muscle coordination and muscle weakness
- ringing in the ears
- dizziness and loss of balance
- slowed or erratic reflexes
- irritability and confusion
- anxiety and depression (neuro-psychiatric)

Pernicious anemia is caused by vitamin B-12 deficiency.

Vitamin B-12 (Cobalamin) is an important vitamin that plays an essential role in the development of the red blood cells. In some countries were their diet is inadequate through low intake of foods rich in vitamin B-12, such as liver, meats and dairy products, they are at higher risk for developing pernicious anemia. The low state of vitamin B-12 is often caused by an autoimmune process.

In the U.S., poor diet is a less common cause. The highest percent of cases in the U.S. are caused by an autoimmune process, whereby the immune system turns on a natural substance in our digestive system and destroys it, rendering it incapable of absorbing proper amounts of vitamin B-12 from the foods we eat.

Foods that are Rich in Vitamin B12

• Clams, Oysters, and Mussels
• Liver
• Caviar (Fish Eggs)
...

...

- Octopus
- Fish
- Crab and Lobster
- Beef
- Lamb
- Cheese (Swiss, Mozzarella, Parmesan, Feta)
- Eggs

This essential vitamin is absorbed by our bodies from the foods we eat, through the digestive system via a substance our bodies produce called "intrinsic factor", a protein that allows for this absorption process to take place. In some people, especially those who have autoimmune diseases, the body will begin to create "antibodies" (killer cells from the immune system), directed against intrinsic factor. Over time, these antibodies begin to destroy this substance and the body will eventually have inadequate amounts for absorbing vitamin B-12 from our diet. People who already have disorders – such as autoimmune thyroid disease, Addison's disease (adrenal glands), lupus, rheumatoid arthritis and other autoimmune disorders – are at higher risk for developing pernicious anemia.

When vitamin B12 levels drop to levels that are below normal, the red blood cells in the body begin to weaken and change size and the number of them diminishes to inadequate levels as well. This is a description of "Pernicious anemia".

Pernicious anemia is treated by replacing the low vitamin B-12 level.

When a doctor confirms that a person has becomes anemic, blood tests for the cause of the anemia will then be conducted. If the cause is found to be low B-12 levels, the treatment prescribed will be to replace the low vitamin and get it back to a normal level.

Most patients are given vitamin B-12 injections to replenish their low levels and they may need an injection administered on a regular schedule, such as once-monthly, for the rest of their lives.

Other patients may take B-12 orally in the form of tablets or liquid, as long as they do not have sensitivity to the oral form of vitamin B-12.

It was once believed that injections were the only method of replacement, but recent medical research articles published on the "PubMed" medical research website state that oral B-12 in sufficiently high amounts can also successfully treat B-12 deficiency. Some doctors might also administer an iron supplement to their patients in addition to replacement of their low B-12 level.

Blood testing of the B-12 levels is the most definitive test for pernicious anemia.

Patients can confirm anemia through a "Complete Blood Count" blood test (CBC), but the test that definitively diagnoses pernicious anemia is a blood test of the vitamin B-12 level. Blood testing labs have normal ranges/values that vary, but if a lab has for example, a normal range for vitamin B-12 of between "200 to 1200 pg/ml" and the patient's result comes back as 150 pg/ml, this would indicate B-12 deficiency as the cause of the anemia. Some blood testing labs make note of the fact that low-normal B12 levels can actually begin to cause symptoms, even before anemia is present. This would be results that are in the range of about 200 to 400 pg/ml which is referred to as "insufficiency" rather than deficiency.

Other vitamins that can cause anemia when they are deficient are folate (vitamin B9) and Vitamin C and blood tests of these should be included if a nutritional cause of anemia is suspected. There is also a blood test to detect antibodies against the protein called intrinsic factor, and if this test comes back positive for these antibodies, this will reveal to the patient and to their doctor that the pernicious anemia is caused by an autoimmune process in the body (digestive tract).

CHAPTER FIVE:

Other Symptoms of Nutritional Deficiencies

The following list describes symptoms for vitamin, mineral and electrolyte deficiencies. Some in the list are in more than one of these three categories. With many of the symptoms being in-common for deficiencies of many of these, diagnostic tests are usually required to definitively determine which nutrient is deficient. Blood lab testing is the most accurate method for detecting these however, "hair mineral analysis", "urine analysis" and "saliva analysis" are also sometimes used, depending on the levels of which type of nutrient is being tested. (Note B12 deficiency symptoms are not included since these were covered in the previous chapter.)

Vitamin A Deficiency - tiredness, stunted growth, insomnia, thick oily skin, immune dysfunction, night vision impairment, weight loss, dry hair

Vitamin C Deficiency - irritability, joint pain, tooth loss, fatigue, gum disease, depression, easy bruising, slowed wound healing

Diagnosing & Treating Common Nutritional Deficiencies

Vitamin D Deficiency - anxiety, osteomalacia (soft bones), bone loss, rickets (bone deformity in children), excessive sweating, burning or tingling sensations in mouth, diarrhea, inability to sleep, nearsightedness

Vitamin E Deficiency - slowed reflexes, lost sense of position, lost sense of vibration, loss of red blood cells, unsteady gait

Vitamin K Deficiency – inability for blood to clot, excessive bleeding

Biotin (B7) Deficiency – clumsiness in muscles, insomnia, myopathy, skin rash and dryness, opthalmopathy, hair that falls out

Calcium Deficiency - depression, inability to sleep, irritability, bone loss, heart arrhythmias, periodontal disease, rickets, tooth loss, dry nails, stomach cramps, hysteria and hallucinations

Chromium Deficiency - glucose dysregulation, type II diabetes, anxiety, fatigue

Copper Deficiency - depression, diarrhea, tiredness, brittle bones, hair that falls out, hyperthyroidism, weak muscles, anemia, arterial artery damage

Deficiencies of Essential Fatty Acids - immune dysfunction, inability to conceive, low sperm count, slowed wound healing, heavy menstrual cycles and PMS, acne, rash and dry skin, gall bladder stones, liver damage, diarrhea, brittle hair and hair loss

Folic acid (B9) Deficiency - headaches, inability to sleep, low appetite and weight loss, fetal deformity, psychosis, breathing difficulties, muscle weakness, anemia, low mood and apathy, diarrhea, tiredness

Iron Deficiency - depression, vertigo, tiredness, headaches, sore tongue, mouth sores, anemia, brittle nails, dementia, constipation

Magnesium Deficiency - hyperactivity, inability to sleep, nervousness, muscular dysfunction and myopathy, restlessness, weakness, anxiety, dementia, heart disease

Manganese Deficiency - hypercholesterolemia, glucose intolerance, hearing problems, clumsy muscles, tinnitus, atherosclerosis, dizziness and vertigo

Niacin (B3) Deficiency - diarrhea, mood disorder, tiredness, irritability, weight loss and loss of appetite, short-term memory loss, myopathy, nausea, skin lesions and dermopathy, bad breath, canker sores, confusion, depression, dermatitis

Pantothenic acid (B5) Deficiency - hair loss, immune impairment, insomnia, irritability, hypotension, muscle cramps, nausea, lack of coordination, abdominal cramps, peripheral neuropathy in feet, depression, eczema, tiredness

Potassium Deficiency - tiredness, hyperglycemia, elevated cholesterol, insomnia, dementia, myopathy, anxiety, hyporeflexia, oily skin, constipation, depression, edema, excessive thirst

Pyridoxine (B6) Deficiency - tiredness, slowed wound healing, irritability, low appetite, hair loss, mouth sores, nausea, acne, anemia, joint pain, opthalmopathy, depression, dizziness, oily face

---

Diagnosing & Treating Common Nutritional Deficiencies

Deficiency in vitamin B6 is fairly rare but can occur in cases of chronic alcoholism.

Riboflavin (B2) Deficiency – peripheral neuropathies (numb hands or feet, loss of sensation, shock or vibration sensations), seizure, eye-sensitivity to light, insomnia and tiredness, weakness, blurry vision, cataracts, low mood, dry-inflamed skin, dizziness and vertigo, hair falling out, eye inflammation, mouth sores, nervousness and irritability

Selenium Deficiency - pancreatitis, indigestion, immune dysfunction, liver dysfunction, low sperm count, stunted growth, elevated cholesterol, increased risk of cancer

Thiamin (B1) Deficiency - low appetite and weight loss, loss of short-term memory, anxiety, peripheral neuropathy, increased pain sensitivity, lack of coordination, weak muscles, dementia, constipation, indigestion, irritability (Deficiency of this vitamin is also called "beriberi disease" but is rare with exception to countries that eat polished rice almost exclusively.)

Zinc Deficiency - elevated cholesterol, immune dysfunction, erectile dysfunction, irritability, malaise, low appetite, lack of ability to taste, low stomach acid (hypochlorhydria), low sperm count, short-term memory loss, partial loss of nighttime vision, psychosis, white areas in the middle of fingernails, slowed wound healing, acne, amnesia, malaise, dry hair and nails, delayed puberty, depressed mood, diarrhea, dry skin rashes, tiredness, stunted growth, loss of hair

Iodine Deficiency – under-active thyroid gland, weight gain, cretinism (neonatal and congenital hypothyroidism), tiredness, joint and muscle aches

Iodine Deficiency Hypothyroidism

I want to add more detail in regard to under-active thyroid gland conditions that occur with iodine deficiency, with hypothyroidism being one of the most common endocrine diseases that exists worldwide. One common acquired type of hypothyroidism that occurs in countries in which their diets are low in iodine is referred to as "iodine deficiency hypothyroidism".

This type is rare in industrialized countries, so is more common in those considered to be "third world countries" (less developed and less industrialized) and is characterized by large goiters (thyroid gland swelling).

You don't often hear of people getting their iodine levels checked because iodine doesn't necessarily tell you anything about your thyroid function. The iodine level in the body can fluctuate due to what is in a person's diet and is influenced by high iodine foods such as kelp or due to supplements one is taking that contain iodine (i.e. a multi-vitamin). The real tests of thyroid function are the actual thyroid hormone levels; "T-4 and T-3" (free levels) and the one called "TSH" which is a pituitary hormone that is sensitive in monitoring thyroid function.

In regard to high iodine content foods or supplements containing iodine, I suggest not consuming these for several days before being evaluated for thyroid function because iodine can work adversely in people with "autoimmune thyroid disease", which is the most common cause of thyroid hormone imbalances in most industrialized countries.

The main form of the disorder being diagnosed is autoimmune thyroiditis – Hashimoto's disease. Iodine is the treatment for hypothyroidism caused by iodine deficiency but this type is almost non-existent in the more advanced countries due to our use of iodized table salt, found in many manufactured foods. Use of iodized salt alone usually contains as much iodine as average, healthy people need for proper thyroid function.

CHAPTER SIX

Diagnostic Testing for Vitamin, Mineral and Electrolyte Imbalances

Ask your Doctor to Order Blood Tests

This is an area that some people may see as unnecessary patient involvement, however, being proactive in your own lab testing and health care through self-education and informed consultations with your doctor can result in a higher quality of care. Doctors are not perfect and they cannot feel in your body what you do. They can treat you according to your symptoms but even this requires detailed input by the patient. If you have come across information online, through reputable medical sources that you feel is significant in regard to your case (i.e. blood tests needing ordered), you need to discuss this with your doctor.

I will admit, personally, that I have been to doctors who were opposed to any input from me as the patient and they were also opposed to my learning about my illness on fellow patient forums or reputable medical websites.

Diagnosing & Treating Common Nutritional Deficiencies

Others have actually appreciated my pro-activeness because it helped them to better optimize my treatment. The U.S. National Institutes of Health has a radio campaign that actually encourages patients to be more informative with their doctors and to ask them questions. The attitude of a doctor in this area may also help you decide whether he is the doctor for you or if you need to seek one who allows more cooperation from you.

Medical blood lab testing is the single most valuable diagnostic testing that is available. Without blood testing, many diseases and disorders, including thyroid hormone disorders would be much more difficult for medical professionals to diagnose.

Understanding your Blood Lab Results

Certainly a patient cannot assume a diagnosis from reading their own blood lab results but requires a licensed medical professional. They can however learn how to basically interpret them, as to whether a result is normal or abnormal and if outside of normal values, how far outside of the range the result is.

Basically understanding blood tests results can help a patient to better discuss them with their doctors.

All lab results have a column beside the title/name of the test that lists your "result" and there will also be a column that lists the "reference range" or "normal values" for each test. When you compare your result to the reference range, this will tell you where your result falls within the normal range or outside of it. Most lab results that fall outside the normal values are "flagged" as abnormal or are highlighted. The lab result page will either have an abnormal column for which to list the flagged results or they will have a notation beside the result such as "L" (meaning low) and "H" (meaning high).

Even results that are within the normal values are not always acceptable as being in a healthy range because with some tests, a borderline high or low level (on the edge of becoming abnormal) indicates the need for close observation and follow-up evaluations.

Diseases, such as borderline diabetes and sub-clinical hormone deficiencies for example, are results that usually need to be followed up on (to monitor for possible development of full-blown disease).

If you do not understand what an abnormally high or low result on particular medical tests means, your doctor should help to inform you about them but you may also want to do a search on the Internet using the name of the blood test as the search term. You will find medical lab websites that will inform you as to what an abnormally high or abnormally low result means and many of the major blood testing labs offer this general information online.

While some people may view this is a form of self-diagnosis or self-treatment, this is not the case because doctors are sometimes limited in their time for informing patients thoroughly about their health disorders and patients need a basic understanding of what an abnormal result may mean for them.

Gaining an understanding of a health disorder versus attempting to treat one, are not the same thing. True medical disorders and diseases require professional attention by a licensed physician and patients do not have the ability to obtain treatments that can only be obtained through prescriptions provided by medical doctors.

Doctors often have time limited to administering treatments, without passing much information on to the patient about their illness, due to increasing numbers of patients and doctor-shortages. It should be recognized that patients have a right to know what is affecting their lives and health. Simply gaining some basic understanding about their illness will not take away from the fact that they will still need a licensed physician to treat them and to prescribe the medications needed.

If you suspect that you or a loved one has or is developing a nutritional deficiency or if a health disorder has developed that can lead to eventual deficiencies in nutrients, it is essential that medical evaluation is sought as soon as possible. Potential damage to systems in the body can occur if diagnosis and treatment is delayed.

It is my hope that this book has provided a good general educational resource on the subject of maintaining and if possible, optimizing nutritional health to prevent illness and to maintain an improved quality-of-life!

(About the Author Follows - Next Page)

ABOUT THE AUTHOR

I am a husband, father, grandfather and lifetime contract salesman, with experience in health writing that began in 2004. I completed theological studies with Liberty University in 1996. I formerly served as editor and forum moderator of Thyroid Health for a major multi-topic content site and as a general health writer for another, where I received 4 Editor's Choice Awards for my articles on health subjects.

In 2003 I was diagnosed with hypothyroidism; "Hashimoto's thyroiditis" being the cause. This autoimmune form of thyroid disease that causes destruction of the thyroid gland resulted in my also developing "Chronic Fatigue Syndrome", due to a compromised immune system with severe co-morbid "Adrenal Fatigue". I also suffered severe anxiety symptoms, including panic attacks early into the onset of Hashimoto's thyroiditis (Hashitoxicosis). A common heart murmur I was diagnosed with in my teens called "Mitral Valve Prolapse", also worsened in severity of symptoms, with the development of these other health disorders.

My eventual receiving of diagnoses was a difficult process with proper diagnostic testing not being ordered by the first doctors I sought treatment from. These types of issues were inspiration for me to become proactive in my own health care and to self-educate myself on these health disorders, which I have done extensively since 2003. I now enjoy sharing this information with other patients experiencing my same health disorders.

(END)